Dementia Dynamics

A Caregiver's Guide for Peaceful Care

by

Lance G. John

Table of contents

Introduction

As morning approaches and the world wakes to the soft buzz of life, a quiet voyage takes place behind the walls of innumerable houses. It is a trip that starts quietly, with the awareness that the road ahead will need patience, understanding, and genuine love. This is the journey of a caregiver for someone with dementia, one that millions of people find themselves on, sometimes unexpectedly, as they become the anchor in the lives of individuals who formerly set the course for them.

Dementia, a name that often conjures up ideas of forgetfulness and confusion, is much more than a simple loss of memory. It is a complicated disorder that affects both the person and others around them. It is a voyage into the very fabric of human connection, testing the connections of relationships as caretakers attempt to preserve the essence of their loved ones amidst the ebb and flow of memories. Dementia is weaved with threads of various colors, each reflecting a particular kind, symptom, and causes. Alzheimer's disease, which gradually erodes memory; vascular dementia, which appears suddenly after a stroke; Lewy body dementia, which causes haunting hallucinations; and frontotemporal dementia, which alters personality and language—all of these forms combine to form a mosaic that is as diverse as it is challenging.

Caregiving is similar to leading a symphony. Each day offers a new movement, a new challenge, necessitating a careful balance of the known and unknown. The caregiver develops the ability to be a maestro, instinctively understanding when to intervene with aid and when to back off to allow for autonomy. It's a give-and-take dance, and it takes both technique and passion to execute.
Throughout this trip, words often fall short, and compassion serves as the lingua franca. It is a language spoken via the caregiver's gaze, touch, and physical presence. It may be found in modest acts of

kindness, soft reassurances, and quiet sacrifices
done for the sake of love and responsibility.
Have it in mind that you are not on this part alone.
There is a community of caregivers, a fellowship of
like-minded people who appreciate the depth of your
dedication and the power of your love. We may
traverse the complexity of dementia together,
finding comfort in one another's experiences and
bravery in our collective expertise.

Dementia is a word that refers to a wide range of
cognitive impairments, a collection of symptoms
that have a major influence on memory,
communication skills, and everyday activities. It is
not a singular sickness, but rather a non-specific
condition affecting millions of individuals
throughout the globe. Understanding dementia is
critical not just for persons who have it, but also for
their families, caregivers, and society as a whole.

The human brain, a natural wonder, is a
sophisticated network of neurons and synapses that
control all thoughts, actions, and memories. When
dementia enters the picture, the network seems to
unravel at the edges. The connections that once fired

quickly and precisely begin to weaken, resulting in the signs of dementia.

Dementia may take various forms, each with its own set of challenges.

Dementia has a dramatic influence on everyday living. Simple things that were once second nature become difficult problems. Familiar people may seem like strangers, and home may feel exotic. Not only do persons with dementia experience bewilderment and irritation, but so do their loved ones.

Caregivers play a crucial role in the lives of people living with dementia. They become memory keepers, the quiet amid the storm, and, in many cases, unsung heroes. Their path is one of patience, love, and, at times, pain, as they see the person they once knew transform before their eyes.

Understanding dementia is a process that starts with awareness and education. It includes learning about the condition, detecting the symptoms, and knowing when to seek assistance. It is about providing a supportive atmosphere that values the dignity and humanity of individuals impacted.

There is presently no treatment for dementia, although research is progressing. Scientists are delving into the complexities of the brain in order to discover the causes of this illness. Medications may alleviate symptoms, and treatments can enhance quality of life, but the actual goal is to find a solution that will return the brains and memories of individuals afflicted.

Hope resides in scientific discoveries, the power of awareness, and the strength of communities banding together to help individuals impacted by dementia. It is found in the experiences of caretakers, the tenacity of families, and the bravery of individuals who live with the illness every day.

Chapter 1

What is Dementia

Dementia is not one illness. It is a broad phrase used to describe a set of symptoms that people may encounter if they have a range of conditions, including Alzheimer's disease. Diseases classified as "dementia" are caused by aberrant brain alterations.

Dementia refers to a group of disorders that impact memory, thinking, and capacity to function on a daily basis.

The condition worsens with time. It mostly affects elderly individuals, however not everyone will get it as they age.

Factors that enhance the likelihood of acquiring dementia include:

- Age (more prevalent among individuals 65 and older)
- High blood pressure (hypertension).
- High blood sugar (diabetes).
- Being overweight or obese, and smoking.
- Too much alcohol consumption,inactivity, social isolation, and depression.

Dementia is a phenomenon produced by a variety of illnesses that gradually kill nerve cells and harm the brain, often resulting in loss in cognitive function (i.e. the capacity to process ideas) that exceeds what would be anticipated from the normal effects of biological aging. While awareness is unaffected, cognitive function impairment is often accompanied, and sometimes preceded by, changes in mood, emotional control, behavior, or motivation.

Dementia has physical, psychological, social, and economic consequences not just for dementia patients, but also for their caregivers, families, and society as a whole. Dementia is often misunderstood and stigmatized, creating hurdles to diagnosis and treatment.

A person with dementia has two or more of these particular issues, including a deterioration in:

- Memory.

- Reasoning.

- Language.

- Coordination.

- Mood.

- Behavior.

Infections or illnesses may damage the regions of your brain that control learning, memory, decision-making, and language, causing dementia to develop.

Dementia symptoms cause a significant deterioration in thinking capabilities, also known as cognitive capacities, that impairs everyday living and independent function. They also influence behavior, emotions, and relationships.

Alzheimer's disease accounts for 60–80% of cases. Vascular dementia, caused by microscopic bleeding and blood artery obstruction in the brain, is the second most frequent kind of dementia. Mixed dementia occurs when various forms of dementia cause brain abnormalities at the same time. There are several additional illnesses that may produce cognitive impairment but are not dementia, some of which are treatable, such as thyroid disorders and vitamin shortages.

Who develops dementia?
Dementia is classified as a late-life illness since it mostly affects the elderly population.

Dementia affects 5% to 8% of all adults over the age of 65, and the incidence increases every five years. It is believed that up to half of adults 85 and older have dementia.

The number of persons aged 65 and over who have Alzheimer's disease and associated dementias by race is:

- Blacks: 14%.
- Hispanics: 12 percent.
- Non-Hispanic whites: 10%.
- American Indians and Alaska Natives: 9 percent
- Asian and Pacific Islanders: 8 percent

How frequent is dementia?

Alzheimer's and associated dementia affect an estimated 5 million Americans aged 65 and more, according to the Centers for Disease Control and Prevention (CDC). The CDC estimates that by 2060, about 14 million individuals will have dementia, accounting for 3.3% of the population.

Alzheimer's disease is the sixth cause of death in the United States, and the fifth leading cause of death among Americans aged 65 and over.

Is memory loss indicative of the onset of dementia?

A widespread misconception concerning memory loss is that it invariably indicates that you or a loved one has dementia. There are several reasons for memory loss. Memory loss alone may not guarantee a diagnosis of dementia.

It is also true that certain memory alterations are normal as we age (some neurons in the brain die naturally). However, this sort of memory loss is not functionally debilitating, which means that it does not interfere with everyday activities.

Dementia impairs your capacity to function. Dementia is not the same as forgetting where you put your keys. A person with dementia may forget what the keys are for.

Common Forms of Dementia

1. Alzheimer's disease.

Alzheimer's disease is the leading cause of dementia in the UK. Early signs may include difficulties with memory, thinking, language, or perception.

Symptoms of Alzheimer's illness

Alzheimer's disease affects people differently. However, there are certain similar first symptoms:

- Memory difficulties.
- Difficulty with thinking and reasoning.
- Symptoms may include linguistic difficulties, alterations in perception, and emotional disturbances.

The signs of Alzheimer's disease will worsen with time. As Alzheimer's disease develops, a person will need more assistance with daily functioning.

What causes Alzheimer's Disease?

Alzheimer's disease is caused by a complicated combination of factors, one of which is the accumulation of two chemicals in the brain known as amyloid and tau. When circumstances in the brain are not optimal, they cluster together to create microscopic formations known as plaques and tangles. These impair the brain's ability to function normally.

Over time, the condition causes particular components to shrink. It also limits the quantity of essential molecules required to transport signals across the brain.

Eventually, the brain struggles to deal with the damage, and the individual has memory and cognitive difficulties. Dementia occurs when these issues make it difficult for the individual to execute ordinary things that they used to accomplish readily.

Being diagnosed with Alzheimer's illness

Anyone who is experiencing worsening memory or cognitive issues should see a health practitioner, usually their GP. If a GP believes the person's symptoms are caused by dementia, they will send them to a local memory service for a more thorough evaluation.
A skilled health expert is typically responsible for diagnosing Alzheimer's disease. Getting an early diagnosis offers several advantages.

Other Types of Alzheimer's Disease

Some less prevalent kinds of Alzheimer's disease do not initially produce memory issues. These are referred to as 'atypical' Alzheimer's. There are four major categories, each with distinct early symptoms:

1. One mostly affecting language, termed logopenic aphasia.
2. Posterior cortical atrophy is one that causes difficulty with seeing and determining where items are in relation to one other.
3. Frontal variants are those that impact behavior and/or thinking. Alzheimer's disease.
4. Corticobasal syndrome is a condition that causes issues with movement, feeling, thinking, perception, and language.

2. Vascular Dementia

Vascular dementia is the second most prevalent kind of dementia. Common early warning symptoms include difficulty planning and focusing, as well as brief episodes of abrupt bewilderment.

Symptoms of vascular dementia

The most prevalent signs of vascular dementia in its early stages are:

1. Difficulties with planning or organizing, making choices, or addressing issues.

2. Problems following a succession of steps (for example, while making a meal).
3. Slower mental speed might lead to difficulty focusing and brief spells of disorientation.
4. A person in the early stages may also have issues with memory and speaking.

Symptoms may appear rapidly or gradually. As vascular dementia advances, the symptoms worsen and pose difficulties with daily life.

Different types of vascular dementia

Vascular dementia is classified into numerous forms, which include:

- Multiple-infarct dementia
- Subcortical Vascular Dementia
- Stroke-related dementia.

They are all caused by difficulties with blood flow to areas of the brain, which subsequently get damaged.

Diagnosing Vascular dementia

Anyone who often has issues with their thinking or memory should see their doctor.
Dementia is often diagnosed by a series of tests conducted by a skilled health expert.
If the symptoms turn out to be dementia, receiving an early diagnosis offers several advantages.

Causes of Vascular dementia.

There are several factors that raise a person's risk of getting vascular dementia. For example, consider their age, any medical issues, and lifestyle choices.

These are referred to as 'risk factors', and some of them may be avoided.
Age is the most significant risk factor for vascular dementia, and the risk rises after 65.

3. Dementia with Lewy Bodies

Dementia with Lewy bodies (DLB) is a kind of dementia caused by Lewy bodies, protein aggregates found in brain cells.

What is dementia with Lewy bodies?

A variety of disorders that damage the brain may produce dementia. Lewy body dementia is caused by Lewy body disease.
In this condition, small protein clumps known as Lewy bodies form in the brain's nerve cells. Lewy bodies was named after FH Lewy, the German doctor who discovered them.

Lewy bodies generate a variety of symptoms, some of which are shared with Alzheimer's disease and others with Parkinson's disease. For this reason, DLB is often misdiagnosed. DLB affects around one out of every ten patients with dementia.

What are the causes of dementia with Lewy bodies?
It is not yet understood why Lewy bodies form in the brain or how they cause dementia. However, we do understand that Lewy body disease:

- Can produce various symptoms. The accumulation of defective proteins in different sections of the brain may lead to reduced quantities of essential chemicals required for message transmission, as well as

the breakdown of nerve cell connections and final cell death.
- Typically develops over a long period of time, generally when a person is becoming older. Lewy bodies may grow in the brain for a long period before symptoms appear.

Having Lewy body disease does not imply that a person's dementia is only caused by the accumulation of Lewy bodies in the brain.

Many DLB patients have an accumulation of additional proteins that cause Alzheimer's disease. This is frequent among adults over the age of 80. Dementia symptoms are often more severe and worsen faster in patients who have both DLB and Alzheimer's.

Parkinson's disease.
Parkinson's disease is also caused by an accumulation of Lewy bodies in the brain. DLB has several symptoms in common with Parkinson's disease. Both present issues with:

Think about movement, emotion, and physical function.

In DLB, dementia symptoms appear before or around the time the individual develops mobility issues.

For persons with Parkinson's disease, dementia symptoms can appear several years after the movement issues begin.

Who develops dementia with Lewy bodies?

Around 5% of patients with dementia are classified as having DLB, however there is strong evidence that the disorder is underdiagnosed. Scientists believe DLB might account for up to 20% of all dementia.

Dementia with Lewy bodies affects males and women almost equally. DLB, like most other varieties of dementia, becomes more frequent after age 65. It may also impact younger individuals. There is no evidence that anything we may be exposed to during our life affects our chance of DLB. A catastrophic head injury (or repeated traumas) may raise the likelihood of getting Parkinson's disease later in life, however it is unclear if this applies to DLB.

Almost all patients with DLB have a sporadic version, which implies the underlying cause is unclear. Certain genes may raise the likelihood of getting DLB.

4. Frontotemporal dementia.
Frontotemporal dementia, sometimes known as 'Pick's disease,' is a less frequent kind of dementia. Early indications sometimes include personality and behavior abnormalities, as well as linguistic challenges.
Frontotemporal dementia (FTD) is a less prevalent kind of dementia. The earliest visible indications of FTD include personality and behavior abnormalities, as well as linguistic problems.

Dementia refers to a set of symptoms that may include memory, thinking, or language impairments, as well as changes in mood, emotions, and behavior. It occurs when the brain is harmed by illness.

The term 'frontotemporal' alludes to the two sets of lobes (frontal and temporal) in the brain that are affected in this kind of dementia. FTD develops when a disease affects nerve cells in these lobes.

This causes the connections between them and the rest of the brain to break down. The amounts of chemical messengers in the brain likewise decrease with time. These messengers enable nerve cells to communicate with one other and the rest of the body.

There are two major kinds of frontotemporal dementia:

- Behavioral variation. FTD is characterized by impairment to the brain's frontal lobes, which mostly causes behavioral and personality issues. These lobes, located below the forehead, process information that influences our behavior and emotional regulation. They also aid in the planning, problem-solving, and sustained attention required to complete a job.
- Primary progressive aphasia (PPA) is caused by injury to the temporal lobes on either side of the brain closest to the ears, resulting in language impairments. This area of the brain serves several functions. The left temporal lobe plays an important role in storing word meanings and item names. Most individuals

rely on their right temporal lobe to
distinguish familiar persons and items.
The earliest visible indications of FTD include
changes in personality and behavior, as well as
linguistic impairments.

These are very distinct from the early signs of more
frequent kinds of dementia. For example, with
Alzheimer's disease, early alterations often result in
issues with daily remembering. Many persons with
early FTD may recall recent events.

What are the signs of frontotemporal dementia?

Frontotemporal dementia affects people differently.
Its symptoms vary greatly and are determined by
which parts of the frontal and temporal lobes are
destroyed, as well as the person's kind of FTD.

FTD, like other types of dementia, progresses over
time. This implies that the symptoms may be
moderate at first, but will worsen with time.

5. Mixed Dementia

Alzheimer's disease and vascular dementia account for the majority of mixed dementia cases. Other dementia combinations are conceivable, including Alzheimer's disease and dementia with Lewy bodies.

Mixed dementia is a disorder in which a person has many types of dementia. Alzheimer's disease and vascular dementia are the most frequent forms.Other dementia combos are also conceivable, including Alzheimer's disease and dementia with Lewy bodies.

At least one out of every ten patients with dementia has been diagnosed with several types. Mixed dementia is far more frequent in older age groups, particularly those over 75.

Despite the fact that many older persons have Alzheimer's disease and vascular difficulties, only a small number are diagnosed with mixed dementia'. Doctors often use the term'mixed dementia' when a person exhibits evident clinical signs of two different diseases that directly contribute to dementia symptoms.

What are the signs of mixed dementia?
The symptoms of mixed dementia differ depending on the kind of dementia present. Often, one kind of dementia predominates over another. In such instances, we refer to this kind as 'predominant'.

Common forms of mixed dementia

Mixed dementia is sometimes caused by a mixture of three different kinds of dementia-causing diseases. However, most diagnoses are a combination of two categories. Here, we will look at two frequent kinds of combined dementia: Alzheimer's disease and vascular dementia, and Alzheimer's disease and Lewy body disease.

6. Young-onset dementia
When someone gets dementia before the age of 65, this is referred to as 'young-onset dementia'. Early indications are more likely to include changes in behavior, language, eyesight, or personality rather than memory loss.
Obtaining an appropriate diagnosis is critical, but it may take longer for a younger individual.

Receiving a young-onset dementia diagnosis

Obtaining an accurate and prompt diagnosis of dementia is crucial. However, for younger individuals, it may take considerably longer. There may be particular causes for this, including:

Young-onset dementia is uncommon, and health practitioners may have little experience correlating the symptoms in a younger individual.
Early symptoms may be difficult to detect or not noticeable. They might be attributed to other things such as stress, difficulty with relationships or employment, or menopause.
This might be because early indications include changes in behavior, language, eyesight, or personality rather than memory loss.
If the younger person with dementia or others disregard early and mild symptoms or attribute them to other reasons, the individual may not get the necessary assistance. It is frequently only after a diagnosis that someone and others around them can reflect on when things began to change.

Understanding the many varieties of dementia is essential for diagnosis, treatment, and care planning.

Each kind has unique issues that need specific assistance and management strategies. Recognizing the distinct characteristics of each kind of dementia allows caregivers and medical experts to better meet the needs of individuals afflicted, providing hope and enhancing quality of life.

Chapter 2

Recognizing Symptoms

Dementia may develop gradually, with symptoms that are readily overlooked or ascribed to normal aging. It is critical to differentiate between sporadic forgetfulness and the chronic, increasing memory loss associated with dementia.

- Memory Loss That Interrupts Daily Life: Forgetting newly learned facts, crucial dates, or events; asking for the same information again.
- Difficulties with Planning or Problem Solving: Difficulties sticking to a plan, dealing with figures, or following a tried-and-true recipe.
- Difficulty Completing Familiar Tasks: Having trouble driving to a familiar area, maintaining a budget, or remembering the rules of your favorite game.

As dementia advances, the symptoms worsen and start to interfere with independence.

- Losing track of dates, seasons, and the passing of time, forgetting where they are or how they arrived.
- Difficulty Understanding Visual Images and Spatial Relationships: Difficulty reading, measuring distance, and detecting color or contrast, which may cause issues when driving.

- New Word Problems in Speaking or Writing: Difficulty following or entering a discussion; halting in the midst of a conversation and unsure how to proceed.

Dementia may also cause changes in behavior and psychological state, which are among the most difficult symptoms for caregivers to handle.

- Withdrawal from job or Social Activities: As dementia progresses, people may begin to withdraw from hobbies, social activities, job projects, and sports.
- Mood and Personality Changes: Becoming confused, distrustful, melancholy, scared, or nervous; easily upset at home, work, with friends, or in situations outside of their comfort zone.

In its latter stages, dementia may impair bodily coordination and sensory processing.

- Decreased or Poor Judgment: Changes in judgment or decision-making, such as handing significant sums to telemarketers or neglecting grooming or hygiene.

- Misplacing Things and Losing the Ability to Retrace Steps: Placing items in strange locations; losing items and being unable to retrace their steps to locate them.

Early detection of these signs is critical. It enables prompt intervention, which may help control the illness and enhance the quality of life for people afflicted. It also allows people and their families to make future plans, such as care alternatives, living arrangements, and financial and legal concerns.

Unraveling the Causes

Dementia is made up of a complicated web of hereditary connections. Some people have a propensity embedded in their DNA, like a faint message from ancestors long ago. The APOE gene, in its different forms, influences Alzheimer's risk. Families follow lines of forgetting, like fading writing on parchment, wondering whether they, too, will carry the weight of memory deterioration.

Lifestyle choices waltz with dementia, their footsteps echoing down the years. Smoking, the slow-burning waltz companion, damages blood arteries, restricting paths for oxygen and nutrients. A poor diet high in fatty fats and sweets joins the dance, and its rhythm has an impact on brain function. And exercise—the agile dancer—can either wash away poisons or remain stationary.

Age, the lifelong spouse, takes center stage. As the years pass, the chance of dementia increases. The once-agile brain shows signs of wear and tear, with synaptic connections weakening and neurons whispering secrets to the wind. Age is both a witness and an accomplice, witnessing memories fade like sepia pictures exposed to the light.

Brain injuries, like forgotten scars, may influence the progression of dementia. A tumble, a collision, or a battlefield blast—the brain absorbs these shocks, sometimes leaving permanent impressions. Chronic traumatic encephalopathy (CTE), which is often found in sports and military veterans, manifests years later, revealing the brain's concealed damage.

Beyond genes and lifestyle, the environment exerts effect. Air pollution, heavy metals, and pesticides—their gentle hums permeate the brain's passageways. Industrial chemicals swing in the backdrop, like phantom dancers, their effects still being felt. The brain, that fragile ecosystem, reacts to various external cues, adapting or succumbing.

Dementia causes are a multidimensional jigsaw, with each component contributing to the total. It is not a single cause, but rather a symphony of forces working together. Researchers, like detectives, examine the evidence: knotted proteins, restricted arteries, and silent mutations. They look for patterns, linkages, and interventions.

In labs and clinics, the search for answers continues. Clinical trials investigate drugs, lifestyle changes, and new techniques. Biomarkers, like celestial compasses, direct researchers to early detection. The brain, that mysterious realm, reveals its secrets slowly, but hope is on the horizon.
Our daily choices—what we eat, how much we exercise, and the quality of our sleep—can have a substantial impact on our brain health. The

following lifestyle variables may increase the chance of getting dementia:

- Diet: High-saturated fat and sugar diets may raise the incidence of dementia, but Mediterranean diets rich in fruits, vegetables, and healthy fats may be beneficial.
- Physical Activity: Research suggests that regular exercise reduces the risk of cognitive deterioration.
- Sleep: Quality sleep is essential for brain health, and interrupted sleep patterns might increase your chance of developing dementia.

Certain medical problems may also contribute to the development of dementia:

- Cardiovascular Disease: Hypertension and atherosclerosis are two conditions that might raise the chance of developing vascular dementia.
- Diabetes: Poorly managed diabetes increases the risk of dementia owing to its impact on blood vessels and glucose metabolism.
- Depression: There is a complicated link between depression and dementia, with

depression sometimes emerging as an early symptom or risk factor.

Our surroundings, both physical and social, may have a significant influence on our brain health.

- Pollution: Air pollution is associated with an increased risk of dementia.
- Heavy Metals: Lead, mercury, and other heavy metals may cause neurotoxicity, which may lead to dementia.
- Social Engagement: Research suggests that having strong social ties and intellectual stimulation reduces the risk of cognitive deterioration.

Chronic inflammation, a continuous, low-grade immune response, is being identified as a possible risk factor for dementia. Infections, autoimmune responses, and lifestyle choices are all potential causes of inflammation.

Chapter 3

Understanding Behavioral Changes

As a person's dementia advances, they may exhibit behaviors that are difficult for others to comprehend. This may be one of the most challenging elements of living with dementia, for both the person with the disease and those around them.

Changes in conduct are sometimes the first indication that someone has dementia. For some individuals, they appear gradually and might be difficult to detect at first. Others may experience more abrupt shifts.
As dementia advances, you may notice additional changes in the person's conduct, making it harder to manage. Looking at the reasons and recognizing the person's wants might be beneficial.

When a person with dementia exhibits unusual behavior, others may mistake it for a sign of the illness, which is not always the case. It's critical to go beyond the conduct and consider what could be driving it.

There might be particular reasons why a person with dementia is acting differently, such as:

- Their dissatisfaction or concern about how dementia affects them (for example, memory loss or language difficulty)
- Their mental and physical wellness.

Symptoms may include difficulty orienting, difficulty recognising familiar places, lack of contact with others, confusion about their physical surroundings, feelings of being out of control, frustration with others' behavior, and a lack of attention.

Dementia may alter a person's personality and habits, leading to behavioral changes. For example, individuals may no longer be able to perform activities they love or pursue their hobbies without assistance, or they may exhibit signs of sadness.

Knowing the individual - how they respond and cope with situations, their preferences, habits, and history - may help you assist them. For example, if the individual has always been irritable or nervous, dementia may exacerbate their symptoms.

Types of conduct
The person's responsiveness to varied requirements causes their behavior to shift in a variety of ways.

These are often referred to as 'difficult behaviors'. Instead, we refer to them as 'challenging conduct'. It's crucial to realize that the individual isn't attempting to be tough. The behavior may be equally difficult for them and for others who assist them.

- Repetitive behavior
- Trailing, Following, and Checking
- Hide, hoard, and lose things.
- Losing inhibitions.
- Accusing agitation, especially restlessness.
- Aggressive conduct
- Sundowning
- Sleep disruption and waking up at night
- Social withdrawal.

Behavioral changes in dementia may be baffling and upsetting for both the patient and their caretakers.

What Caused the Changes

To decipher behavioral changes, we must first identify their causes. These might be internal, like bodily pain or perplexity, or external, such an overstimulating atmosphere or a disruption in habit.

- Physical Discomfort: Pain, hunger, or the need to use the restroom may all cause agitation.
- Environmental Factors: Loud sounds, clutter, or strange surroundings may all generate anxiety and disorientation.
- Communication Breakdowns: Misunderstandings or an inability to convey demands may be frustrating.

Strategies to Navigate Behavioral Changes

Navigating these changes requires a diverse strategy that includes environmental alterations, communication strategies, and individualized treatments.

- Create a Calm Environment: Simplify living environments, eliminate noise, and stick to a consistent pattern to offer a feeling of security.
- Effective Communication: Use straightforward language and nonverbal clues to connect and reassure. Personalized Activities: To foster a feeling of purpose, engage in meaningful activities that are relevant to the individual's interests and talents.

Empathy, or the capacity to comprehend and share the emotions of others, is crucial to regulating behavioral changes. Caregivers may better anticipate and react to the needs of those suffering from dementia by putting themselves in their place.

- Listen and Observe: Use nonverbal signs and emotional clues to identify underlying requirements.

- Validate Your Feelings Recognize emotions without judgment and validate the individual's experience.
- Adapt and Adjust: Be open to changing tactics as the individual's needs and talents grow.

Chapter 4

Communication Strategies

In dementia care, communication is more than just exchanging words; it is the bridge that links us to the inner worlds of persons we care for. As dementia advances, this bridge may become frail, but with the correct tactics, it may be strengthened with knowledge and compassion.

Communicating with a person with dementia
Dementia is a degenerative disorder that gradually impairs a person's capacity to recall and comprehend fundamental daily information such as names, dates, and locations.
Dementia increasingly affects a person's ability to communicate. Their capacity to articulate reasonable thoughts and reason coherently will change.

If you are caring for someone with dementia, you may discover that as the condition advances, you may need to initiate conversations in order for the individual to communicate. This is common. Their capacity to interpret information gradually deteriorates, and their answers may become delayed.

Encourage someone with dementia to communicate.

Try to initiate talks with the person you're caring for, particularly if you observe that they're having fewer interactions themselves. It can assist with:

- Speak clearly and slowly, using short phrases.
- Make eye contact with the individual while they are speaking or asking inquiries.
- Give them time to react, since they may feel pressured if you attempt to rush their replies.
- Encourage children to participate in talks and allow them to speak out about their own welfare or health concerns.
- Try not to patronize or mock what they say.
- Recognize what they have said, even if they do not answer your question or what they say seems out of context. Demonstrate that you heard them and invite them to elaborate on their response.
- Give them easy options - Avoid making complex choices or alternatives for them.
- Use alternate methods to communicate, such as rephrasing questions since they cannot respond in the same manner they used to.

Communicating with body language and physical touch

Communication is more than simply talking. Gestures, movement, and facial expressions may all communicate meaning or help you get your point across. When a person with dementia struggles to communicate, body language and physical interaction become more important.

When someone is having trouble communicating or comprehending, try:

- Being patient and calm might help the individual communicate more freely.
- Maintain a cheerful and welcoming tone and maintain a reasonable distance to prevent frightening others. Patting or holding someone's hand during a conversation might comfort them and provide a sense of closeness. Watch their body language and listen to what they say to determine whether they're okay with you doing this.
- It is critical that you encourage the individual to articulate their desires in whatever way

they are capable. Remember, we all become frustrated when we can't communicate well or are misunderstood.

Listening to and comprehending a person with dementia
Communication is two-way. As a caregiver for someone with dementia, you will most likely need to improve your listening skills.
You may need to be more attentive of nonverbal cues like facial expressions and body language. You may need to make additional physical contact, such as comforting pats on the arm, or smiling in addition to speaking.

- Active listening may assist.

- When speaking with someone, maintain eye contact and urge them to look at you. Avoid interrupting them, even if you understand what they're saying. Pause your activity to give them your entire attention while they speak.
- To improve communication, avoid distractions like loud TV or radio, but always

verify whether it's okay to do so. Also, repeat what you heard back to the individual and confirm accuracy, or ask them to repeat what they said.

Patience, respect, and empathy are essential components of effective communication with someone suffering from dementia. It entails knowing the individual's background, preferences, and present talents. It's about establishing a place where they feel heard and appreciated, regardless of the difficulties dementia may cause.

As dementia impairs cognitive ability, communication tactics must adjust correspondingly.

The environment has an important influence in communication.

- Reduce Distractions: Remove background noise and visual clutter to assist the individual concentrate on the talk.

- Comfortable Settings: Make sure the individual is comfortable and relaxed, since this might lead to higher participation.
- Consistent Surroundings: Familiar surroundings may help people with dementia feel more safe and orientated, which improves communication.

Active listening is an effective approach in dementia care.

- Pay Full Attention: Maintain eye contact and demonstrate that you are listening. This expresses respect and makes the individual feel understood.
- Be patient: Allow the individual time to express themselves, even if it takes longer than normal.
- Reflect and Clarify: Repeat what you've heard to confirm comprehension and allow the individual to address any misconceptions.

Communication issues are frequent in dementia care, but they may be addressed with creative strategies:

- Repetitive Questions: Respond patiently each time, realizing that the repetition is due to dementia.
- Word-Finding Difficulties: If the individual is having trouble finding words, gently offer them or ask them to express what they're thinking.
- misconceptions: If there are any misconceptions, be cool and comforting. Consider rephrasing your message or addressing the subject from a fresh perspective.

Technology may be an effective communication tool in today's digital age:

- Communication Devices: Tablets and specialized applications may help people

communicate more effectively, particularly those who struggle with language.
- Social Media: Platforms such as Facebook may assist preserve social ties while also providing excitement with photographs and messages from friends and family.

Caregivers might benefit from training and assistance to improve their communication skills.

- Education: Understanding dementia and its influence on communication may help caregivers prepare for the difficulties ahead.
- Support Groups: Sharing your experiences with other caregivers may offer both practical advice and emotional support.
- Professional Guidance: Speech therapists and dementia care professionals may provide personalized methods and treatments.

Chapter 5

Managing Agitation and Aggression.

Some people with dementia may exhibit or suffer agitation and hostility against their family members or caregivers at some time. They may be defined as follows.

Agitation refers to a range of behaviors shown by individuals with dementia who experience anxiety, whether verbal or motor.

Aggression may manifest as verbal abuse, threats, property damage, physical violence, or exaggerated reactions to small setbacks or criticism.

Dementia development may lead to agitation and aggression due to a lack of behavioral control.

Physical discomfort includes pain, fever, sickness, or constipation.

Fatigue caused by a lack of sleep.

When one's independence and freedom are endangered, they engage in defensive conduct.

Frustration stems from an inability to complete everyday chores.

Fear of surroundings or persons because the person with dementia is unable to identify them.

An adverse response to medicine.

Tips for Managing Agitation and Aggression.

Dealing with aggressive behavior is not simple. It is always beneficial to know what causes the hostility and devise efficient techniques to handle it.

It is vital to understand that it might be a form of communication depending on how a person with dementia acts. If we can figure out what he or she is trying to say, it may avoid them from being irritated and angry.

Agitation and violence in dementia may arise from a number of reasons, including irritation with their inability to communicate properly or grasp what is going on around them. Factors that may contribute include:

- Physical Discomfort refers to pain, discomfort, or medical conditions such as infections or constipation.
- Environmental Triggers include overstimulation, loud sounds, or a congested environment.
- Psychological Factors include fear, perplexity, and a sense of being endangered.
- Unmet Needs include hunger, thirst, and the desire for social connection.

Here are several approaches to handle such behavior:

- Identify or become aware of signals or behaviors that indicate agitation or violence. Distract the individual with dementia with suitable activities before his or her outburst.
- Keep harmful materials like scissors, knives, and sharp objects out of the surroundings to ensure its safety.
- Maintain your cool and avoid escalating the situation. A passionate reaction from you may exacerbate the problem.
- Approach your loved one cautiously, comfort him/her, and realize that he/she is sad.
- If the person with dementia becomes agitated/aggressive while you care for him/her,
- Explain your activities in short, basic terms like "I'm going to help you take off your shirt" or "We're here to help you."
- Consider if what you're doing for the other is really necessary at the time.
- Give him or her some time and space before returning to gently try again.
- If the individual with dementia becomes physically aggressive.

- Make some distance between you and the person with dementia (at least one arm's length) to avoid physical harm.
- Do not attempt to contain or restrict the outpouring of anger unless it is causing damage to the individual or others.
- Call for assistance if necessary.
- Ensure your loved one's basic requirements are satisfied, such as hunger, thirst, and enough sleep.
- Try to be consistent in their daily routines, surroundings, and caregivers.
- Ensure that the person with dementia's medical problems and medicines are examined on a regular basis by their doctor.

Nondrug approaches outperform drugs in terms of reducing agitation and hostility in dementia patients. Physical movement, touch and massage, and music are all effective techniques for managing dementia-related agitation.

The environment has an important influence in controlling behaviors.

- Declutter: Keeping your home clean and orderly will help you feel less anxious or agitated.
- Control Noise: Reduce background noise to avoid overstimulation.
- Optimize illumination: Provide appropriate illumination to make the user feel safe and orientated.

Each person is unique, as are their causes for anger and violence.

- Know the Person: Understanding the person's background, likes, and dislikes will help you adjust your approach to their specific requirements.
- Individualized Activities: Participate in activities that the individual enjoys and finds relaxing.
- Personal Space: Respect the individual's need for personal space and privacy.

In certain circumstances, medication may be essential.

- Consult Healthcare Providers: Always seek expert guidance before using medication to treat habits.
- Monitor effects: Be aware of side effects and the influence of drugs on the individual's quality of life.

Managing agitation and aggressiveness in dementia is a complicated endeavor that needs a caring, knowledgeable approach. Understanding the underlying reasons, using appropriate communication skills, and establishing a supportive atmosphere may help caregivers manage these behaviors with confidence and offer the greatest care for their loved ones.

Chapter 6

Overcoming Resistance to Care.

Dementia patients may be aware of their cognitive impairment, but may not fully understand how it impacts their capacity to live freely. Some claim they lack insight. While it may be challenging to keep track of expenses, mailing blank checks in the mail may go unnoticed. Attending social gatherings may be difficult, but individuals may not know they are presenting themselves to the same person. They may believe they can take care of themselves and their home, yet fail to detect outdated food or unwashed clothes.

Inexperienced caregivers may bring out inadequacies to their loved ones with dementia. Reacting with embarrassment, humiliation, denial, confabulation, or stubbornness will simply exacerbate the situation rather than fix it. Everyone is upset. The invoices remain unpaid. The filthy clothes are still in stacks.

Inadequate understanding may lead to resistance to care, unwillingness to acknowledge the need for aid, and rejection to accept help. Caregivers of dementia patients sometimes face resistance to care, particularly during the early and middle phases of the illness.

Resistance to care may take many forms, ranging from blatant denial of aid to subtle avoidance of tasks. It is critical to recognize that this resistance is not a personal assault, but rather a response to the uncertainty, anxiety, and frustration that often precede dementia.

- Loss of Independence: As dementia develops, people may reject receiving care in order to maintain their independence.
- Fear and worry: Routine or environmental changes may cause worry, which leads to resistance.
- Misunderstanding: Cognitive limitations might cause misconceptions regarding the goals behind care efforts.

Dementia patients need support. Whether they accept it or not, this is the reality of the situation. They need assistance. How can a caretaker help someone who refuses to accept help?
Caregivers should improve their communication skills and awareness of dementia. Caregivers must create techniques to address resistance to treatment without insulting or overwhelming patients.

Some techniques that may be helpful:

- Don't argue.Helping someone with a major impairment is more important than being correct.
- Avoid attempting to persuade or explain why they should accept aid since they may not understand logical reasoning.
- Conduct a detailed review of the circumstances behind the denial of treatment. Is it based on previous habits or occurrences from your loved one's earlier years? Dementia may bring back previous behaviors, contrary to popular belief.
- To address a person's resistance, it's important to understand their personal history and identity.
- Consider physical restrictions, such as arthritis, hearing loss, or impaired vision. Remember that individuals with dementia may be unable to communicate their concerns.
- Pick your fights.Is it about safety or personal preferences? Is it essential to wash daily, or might a sponge bath serve in between? Can

you make adjustments to make the activity more pleasurable for them?

- Encourage your loved one to participate in decision-making. While kids may not be able to choose their attire, they can respond to questions like "Do you want the red or blue shirt?"
- Use visual signals instead of verbal ones.A doctor's statement declaring "No driving" may be more helpful than just instructing someone not to drive.
- Be delicate and utilize subtlety.It is not always necessary for individuals to be aware of the assistance they receive. Laundry may be done while out to lunch, mail can be presorted, a caretaker can be engaged like a cleaning lady, and prescription medications can be taken as vitamins.
- Use fiblets or make up a narrative to help them unwind.
- If he doesn't want to go to the doctor, explain that changes in social security now need it. If he insists on driving, explain that the automobile is broken and propose waiting for a replacement component from the retailer.

- Seek the assistance of specialists.Advice from a lawyer, medical, or law enforcement agency may be more credible.
- Create support mechanisms to cope with loss of independence. Connect with transportation services, GPS monitoring systems, and family members to help your loved one remain active and sociable. Contact the Alzheimer's Association for information and solutions.
- Do not give up.You may always try again later or on another day.

In late stages of dementia, caregivers may need to adapt their approach and expectations to accommodate the patient's limits and personal routines, making resistance to care less prevalent. According to studies, just 9% of nursing home residents refuse treatment.
Consult your neurologist if you are experiencing persistent resistance to treatment. Dementia-related anxiety and rejection of care may be reduced using safe and effective drugs.

The surroundings may have a substantial influence on an individual's desire to get treatment.

- Consistent Routine: Maintaining a consistent daily routine might help to lessen anxiety and resistance.
- Personalized areas: Decorate care areas with objects that are personal to the individual, such as pictures or preferred décor.
- Reduce Overstimulation: Maintain a quiet atmosphere by avoiding loud sounds and busy images that might be overpowering.

As dementia develops, the individual's requirements and capacities alter.

- Flexibility: Be prepared to adapt care plans when the patient's condition changes.
- Monitoring Responses: Observe how the person reacts to various approaches and adjust strategies appropriately.
- Professional Input: Seek assistance from healthcare specialists on how to tailor treatment to the individual's changing needs.

Education is an effective method for reducing resistance to care.

- Dementia Training: Educate caregivers and family members on dementia and its impact on behavior.
- Support Groups: Encourage involvement in support groups where people may share their experiences and learn from one another.
- Resource Availability: Make materials accessible that provide advice and approaches for dealing with patient resistance to treatment.

Chapter 7

Designing a Dementia-Friendly Home

Creating a dementia-friendly house entails designing an atmosphere that promotes the well-being and independence of people with dementia. It is a secure, welcoming, and familiar environment in which the problems of dementia are addressed with deliberate design and caring understanding.

How to make your house dementia-friendly.
Your home's design and layout may have a significant influence on someone with dementia. Symptoms of memory loss, disorientation, and trouble learning new things indicate that someone with dementia may forget where they are, where things are, and how they operate.
Although it is not recommended to make big modifications to the house overnight, there are some easy things you may do to assist someone with dementia live freely at home.
1. Needs evaluation.
   If the person with dementia has not already done so, it is critical to get a needs assessment from your local council.
2. Better illumination.
   Most persons with dementia, and older people in general, benefit from improved illumination in their homes, which may assist to prevent confusion and lower the risk of falling.

3. Try to minimize glare, shadows, and
   reflections.

The lighting should be bright, even, and
natural (to the extent feasible). To increase
natural light throughout the day, make sure
that:

- Curtains are open.
- Nothing, including superfluous nets
  and shades, is obscuring the windows.
- Hedges and trees are chopped down if
  they impede the sunlight.
- Lighting is especially vital on the
  stairs and in the toilet. Light switches
  should be simple to reach and operate.

- Automatic light sensors might be
  useful additions. When someone
  passes the sensor, the lights turn on
  automatically.

It is also crucial to ensure that the bedroom is
dark enough at night to aid with sleep.

Because dementia is more frequent among the elderly, annual eye exams are essential for detecting and treating any issues.

4. Reduce excessive noise:
   Carpets, cushions, and drapes reduce background noise. Walking across the room on laminate or vinyl flooring may be quite loud. If the person with dementia uses a hearing aid, the noises will be magnified, which may be unpleasant.
   If no one is watching television or listening to the radio, switch them off.
   Even if the person with dementia wears hearing aids, frequent hearing exams are necessary.

Dementia patients' symptoms might be exacerbated by issues with both sight and hearing.

5. Safer flooring.
   Try to avoid carpets or mats on the floor since some individuals with dementia may get confused and believe the rug or mat is an item they need to walk over, resulting in trips or falls.

Avoid bright or reflective flooring since it may be seen as damp, making it difficult for the person with dementia to walk on.

The finest flooring to choose is matt and in a color that contrasts with the walls. It may be beneficial to avoid using hues that are easily confused for genuine objects, such as green (grass) or blue (water).

6. Contrasting colors
   Dementia may impair someone's ability to distinguish between hues. Choose:

   Decorate using contrasting colors on walls, floors, and furniture, such as beds, tables, and chairs.
   To make items stand out, use contrasting colors for doors and banisters, toilet seats, and tableware to define edges.
   Avoid utilizing strong patterns and stripes, since they may be confusing and disorienting.

7. Reflections may be troublesome.
   Check mirrors and cover or remove any that may create confusion in the dementia patient.

They may get concerned if they do not
identify themselves.
Similarly, closing the curtains in the evening
might assist them to avoid seeing their
reflection in the window glass.

8. Labels and signage may assist people move
   around.
   Labels and signs on cabinets and doors might
   be useful, such as a toilet sign on the
   bathroom or toilet door. The signs should be:

   - To ensure clarity, use clear wording
     and a visually appealing image that
     contrasts with the backdrop. Place the
     image somewhat lower than usual to
     accommodate aging eyes.
   - It may also be beneficial to place
     images on cabinets and drawers to
     indicate what is within them. For
     example, you may display a picture of
     cups on the cabinet that houses them.

Alternatively, see-through cabinet doors may be
quite helpful to someone with dementia since they
allow them to see what is within.

Dementia-friendly home products

There are home goods available that are particularly developed for persons with dementia. For example:

- Features include huge LCD clocks, massive buttons on phones, and auditory reminders to remind individuals to take medications or lock the door.
  These items are typically referred to as assistive technology. Apps for cellphones and tablets are also useful.

- Gardens and outdoor places.
  People with dementia, like everyone else, may benefit from being out in the fresh air and exercising. Ensure that:

  - Walking surfaces are flat to avoid stumbles and falls.
  - Outdoor spaces should be secure to prevent wandering, with raised flower beds to assist those with limited mobility, sheltered seating areas, and adequate lighting. Garden entrances

should also be easily visible and accessible.

☐ Bird feeders and insect boxes will attract wildlife to your yard. A variety of flowers and plants may also help people remain interested.

Chapter 8

The Function of Routine and Structure

Routine and structure in dementia care are more than simply organizational tools; they are the foundations that might support the frail architecture of a fading memory.

Caring for someone with dementia is demanding and hard. Most caregivers are unprepared for the many challenges they will experience on their path of caring. Dementia-related brain changes, including memory loss, may induce worry, anxiety, and illogical conduct. The significance of regularity and familiarity for people with dementia is tremendous! Aggression, restlessness, and agitation are examples of undesirable behaviors that may be reduced by daily routine. As a consequence, the caregiver will be less stressed and better equipped to provide care.

How can daily routine lead to reduced stress?

Daily routines can alleviate stress and anxiety by letting everyone involved know what to anticipate. Individuals with dementia thrive on familiarity. Familiarity is vital since dementia progressively reduces a person's capacity to organize, begin, and finish activities. By providing an atmosphere with familiar habits and activities, they might feel at ease and peaceful. If they can still engage in an activity, they can maintain their feeling of control and independence. Furthermore, creating a familiar sequence of occurrences may aid in the transfer of a daily routine's schedule to the brain's long-term memory.

What should I consider while developing a routine?

If your loved one has cognitive impairment or is in the early stages of dementia, monitor his or her washing, clothing, grooming, eating, and toileting habits. What time of day and where in the home do they occur? Does he or she have a favorite wardrobe item or color? What is his or her favorite cuisine or drink? At this stage of the condition, attentively watching and maintaining them might be useful in the long term. If his or her dementia has progressed to a later stage, attempt to recollect them. The more activities a caregiver may arrange that reflect their loved one's pre-dementia life, the better.

Other familiar hobbies and interests contribute to the caring experience. What genres of music does your loved one appreciate, and more specifically, which songs? Do they have any favorite TV series or movies that they enjoy? What hobbies or leisure activities do he or she enjoy? If you're unsure, make a note of them. The more you can get your loved one involved in these activities, the more safe and comfortable they will feel.

What more could I do?

If you are a caregiver for someone with early dementia, maybe this information will help. It is critical that your loved one work as hard as they can for themselves for as long as possible. Even as the condition advances, it is critical to keep these habits. Eventually, your loved one will need your assistance. If your loved one can still complete certain things with your help, consider doing them together. Doing things on your own may be simpler, but it is not the greatest option.

The goal is to establish a regimen that incorporates activities that are appropriate for your loved one's abilities. In doing so, you'll establish a consistent atmosphere that will provide some comfort and comprehension in an increasingly complicated world. Giving your loved one a day free of surprises is the most effective method to help them expend energy, ease worry, and reduce unpleasant behaviors.

Routine lends a reassuring hand amid the darkness of dementia. It gives regularity in a world that might often seem chaotic and confusing. Here's why routines matter:

- Reduces Stress: Knowing what to anticipate might help people with dementia feel less anxious and stressed.
- Promotes Independence: Familiar routines may help people preserve their skills and independence for as long as feasible.
- Improves Sleep: Maintaining a regular sleep pattern leads to greater sleep quality, which is essential for cognitive health.

Creating a daily schedule requires knowing the individual's life history, preferences, and present skills.

- Consistent Wake-Up Time: Begin each day at the same time to establish a pattern.
- Mealtime Rituals: Serve meals on a regular schedule and, if feasible, include the person in basic preparation.
- Activity Blocks: Set aside regular periods for activities, exercise, and social contact to increase stimulation and engagement.

Structure is the foundation on which procedures are constructed. It's about establishing an environment that's simple to traverse and comprehend.

-
- Distinct Layout: Divide the living area into distinct zones for various activities, such as dining, resting, and personal care.
- Visual cues: Use signs, symbols, or colors to designate distinct locations and help you navigate.
- Familiar things: Place familiar things around your house to act as markers and memory aids.

As dementia advances, the individual's demands vary, and routines must adjust accordingly:

- Flexibility: Be willing to adjust routines to meet changes in abilities and preferences.
- Simplification: Simplify activities and procedures as required to avoid aggravation and achieve success.
- Personalization: Customize routines to the individual's background, such as including

components from their previous job or
interests.

Therapeutic activities should be included into the
everyday routine to improve well-being:

- Music Therapy: Schedule time for listening
  to music, which may be soothing and
  uplifting.
- Art and Crafts: Plan creative activities that
  encourage self-expression and reflection.
- Physical Exercise: Incorporate light exercise
  to help preserve mobility and physical fitness.

A well-established routine may positively affect
behavior.

- Reduces Agitation: Establishing predictable
  routines may help to reduce agitation and
  confusion.
- Reduces Sundowning: Evening rituals may
  help alleviate symptoms of sundowning, such
  as restlessness and agitation.
- Improves Cooperation: When people
  understand what to anticipate, they are more
  inclined to participate in care activities.

Technology may be a great partner in sustaining habits.

- Automated Reminders: Configure devices to provide aural or visual reminders for activities and prescriptions.
- Digital Calendars: Use digital calendars to organize appointments and special occasions.
- Monitoring Systems: Consider implementing monitoring systems to assure safety and regular compliance.

Caregivers also benefit from regularity and structure.

- Self-Care Scheduling: Incorporate self-care activities into the caregiver's daily routine to minimize burnout.
- Professional Development: Set up time for caregivers to attend training and support groups.

- Respite Care: Arrange for frequent respite care to allow caregivers to rest and preserve their well-being.

Chapter 9

Therapeutic Activities and Engagement.

Therapeutic activities, which may range from attending an exercise class to playing a board game to hosting a BBQ with friends and family, can be very beneficial and fulfilling for dementia patients, making them feel happier, more relaxed, and healthier.

Furthermore, consistent participation in therapeutic activities may enhance physical and cognitive function, slowing illness progression, improving quality of life, and enhancing the patient's capacity to carry out everyday chores.

30 therapeutic activities to inspire family members and caregivers when deciding what to do with their loved ones. Whenever feasible, we advocate allowing the patient to pick what they want to do, giving them a feeling of control and significance in how they spend their time.

To make things easier, we've divided the list of activities into the following categories:

1. Physical activities.
2. Cognitive activities.
3. Sensory activities.
4. Creative activities.

How Do Therapeutic Activities Benefit Dementia Patients?

Engaging in meaningful therapeutic activities may help reduce dementia symptoms, enhance patients' quality of life, and guarantee that their basic requirements are satisfied. Activities are also useful in coping with problematic behaviors, assisting caregivers in soothing or distracting patients who are restless or upset. These exercises may benefit individuals in various stages of dementia (early, medium, and late-stage) and kinds (Alzheimer's disease, frontotemporal dementia, Lewy Body dementia, and more).

Overall, therapeutic activities enable patients to:

- A feeling of purpose.
- A method to apply skills and life experiences.
- Benefits include increased self-esteem and the chance to connect with loved ones.
- Benefits include more independence and decision-making opportunities.
- A method for improving physical and cognitive abilities.
- A method for maintaining the capacity to do activities of daily living (ADLs).
- A method to feel more productive.

Factors to Consider When Planning Activities

It might be difficult to come up with new things to undertake on a daily basis while caring for someone who has dementia.

Here are a few suggestions to help you decide:

1. Timing is critical: To gain the best results while carrying out activities, caregivers must consider the time of day when the patient is most aware. For example, some patients may like going for a morning stroll, whilst others may prefer to sit at home with a cup of tea, reminiscing, and browsing through old picture albums. It's also necessary to ensure that the patient isn't concerned about anything. If they are, they will be unable to focus on the work.

2. Activities should be entertaining and interesting. Fun and engaging activities may help lessen disruptive behaviors like frustration and agitation. Ideal activities include music, arts & crafts, and sensory stimulation. Furthermore, people with dementia may enjoy going out for the day, even if they subsequently forget where they

were. What matters is that they had a good time, even if the event will be forgotten quickly.

3. Activities must be exciting: Choosing stimulating activities is critical for keeping people engaged both physically and psychologically. What each patient finds intriguing and engaging will differ. Doing activities that patients have previously enjoyed is a wonderful method to locate the correct ones. For example, if your loved one was an avid gardener, they could still enjoy spending time in their garden. Alternatively, if they have always loved going for a coffee and reading the newspaper in the morning, they may wish to continue doing so even if they are unable to read the whole article. The trick is to find the proper balance: Activities must be exciting enough to keep the patient engaged but not so tough that the patient feels irritated or angry.

4. Activities must be tailored to the patient's ability. As the patient's skills fluctuate during the illness, caregivers must adapt and tweak

activities to match what they can accomplish. For example, patients in the early stages of dementia may participate in difficult cognitive games, but patients in the latter stages may need more soothing activities, such as listening to music. Furthermore, senior individuals may have pre-existing diseases such as heart difficulties, arthritis, or high blood pressure, which may restrict their ability to participate in some activities, particularly those requiring physical exertion.

5. Activities must take place in a secure and pleasant atmosphere, which is especially important for activities done at home. Patients with dementia often have eye issues, including difficulties with visual perception and coordination. To prevent mishaps and falls, make sure all work surfaces are clean and clutter-free, and that the space has enough illumination. Also, while exercising, try to prevent distractions and keep noise to a minimum.

How You Can Help As A Caregiver

Here are some pointers to keep in mind when you engage in dementia activities with your loved one.

1. Help get the activity started: Patients with dementia still want to do things, but they may require assistance with planning and initiating activities.
2. Provide support: Provide as much assistance as required to carry out your tasks. The ideal approach is to give basic, easy-to-follow instructions. Too many directions may be intimidating.
3. Focus on the process, not the outcome: It makes no difference if the table isn't configured correctly. What counts is that your loved one feels helpful while participating in a family activity at home.
4. Be flexible: If your loved one refuses to do anything, don't push it. Similarly, even if the activity does not go as planned, urge them to continue.
5. Assist with the tough aspects of the activity: If you're cooking with a loved one, for example, they may want assistance measuring ingredients or understanding the

instructions. Find a method to assist with the challenging tasks and propose something else they might do instead.

6. Let your loved one know that they are wanted. Throughout the process, ask for your loved one's assistance so that they know they are required.

7. Never criticize or correct your loved ones. Allow your loved one to do the task as they see fit, even if you believe it is the incorrect way. Encourage them to keep going as long as it is safe.

8. Allow self-expression. Include activities in which your loved one may communicate their thoughts and emotions. Painting or listening to music are excellent options for this.

9. Keep the discussion going: Whatever activity you choose, maintain the conversation with your loved one. Even if they are unable to answer (as the sickness worsens), they will still appreciate hearing your voice.

10. Try again later. If anything you planned doesn't work, try again later. It may be the incorrect time of day, or your loved one may be concerned about something.

11. Be encouraging. Encourage your loved one to continue participating in various activities that give mental stimulation.
12. Be prepared to adapt: Always be prepared to modify your scheduled activity as required. Instead of merely listening to music, your loved one may also want to dance.
13. Allow your loved one to choose the activity. When feasible, let the patient pick what they wish to do. They are more inclined to participate in an activity that they choose.

1. Physical activities.

Physical exercise has various advantages for dementia patients, including better cardiovascular fitness, strength, and endurance. It may also help to slow down dementia-related symptoms including cognitive decline and sleep difficulties. Regular physical exercise is critical for preserving patients' independence for as long as feasible.

Regular exercise has several health advantages, including:

- Benefits include improved mood, better sleep, improved motor skills, lower chance of falling, increased strength, and improved balance.
- Improved memory and cognitive skills
- Improved behavior, such as less roaming, cursing, and aggressiveness.
- improved communication and social abilities.
- Lower risk of heart disease and diabetes.
- Reduced stress, increased self-sufficiency and confidence.

Physical exercise may be difficult for older persons, especially those who did not exercise when they were younger. Caregivers may aid by following these safety guidelines:

- Consult with the patient's doctor about the sort of exercise that is appropriate for them, particularly if they have pre-existing diseases that restrict their mobility. Some people may need a comprehensive medical exam.
- Take things gradually. Patients may initially be able to accomplish just five minutes of light exercise, but with time, they will be able to progressively increase their activity.

- Perform the exercise concurrently with the patient. Caregivers may show a set of exercises and instruct the patient to follow.
- Make sure the activity is exciting and engaging. If patients are bored (because it is too easy) or overwhelmed (because it is too tough), they are less likely to be inspired to continue.
- When you're outdoors, ensure the patient is wearing a medical alert bracelet and identification in case they walk away and get lost.
- If the patient is fit enough to chat while exercising, keep the discussion going as long as feasible. This keeps the patient interested while also allowing you to measure their fatigue levels.
- If you're going outside in the summer, make sure the patient wears a hat and applies sunscreen to all exposed skin.
- To prevent dehydration, ensure that the patient drinks lots of water when exercising.
- If the patient complains of dizziness or discomfort, halt the activity.

1. Go on a Walk

Walking is one of the most beneficial workouts for patients, and it is completely free. Furthermore, it may be integrated with other duties that caretakers must do, such as grocery shopping or walking the dog. Walking also helps to regulate certain disruptive behaviors, and patients are less likely to wander away if they know they are going for a stroll.

Patients should walk 4-5 times a week for 30 minutes with short breaks. When this becomes an issue, patients may still go for numerous short walks throughout the day, even if they are just around the garden. Always ensure that the patient is wearing comfortable shoes and lightweight clothing.

2. Go on a bike ride.

Some patients may appreciate going on a bike ride. Even patients in the latter stages of the condition, as long as they do not have balance issues, may enjoy a leisurely bike ride. Caregivers must remain close to patients to prevent them from getting disturbed.

If patients are hesitant to ride alone, tandem bikes enable caretakers to sit in the front and operate the bike while the patient sits in the back and pedals.

3. Exercises for Improving Balance

Patients with dementia often feel dizziness and other balance issues. Balance exercises may lower the risk of falls and help you stay independent for longer. Furthermore, these workouts benefit the vestibular system, strengthen balance-related muscles, increase cognitive function, and make everyday tasks more manageable.

Some possibilities include:

- Leg stances: For safety, stand with both feet together in a corner or against a countertop. For an extra difficulty, place one foot in front of the other in a straight line.
- Rock the Boat: Lean slightly from side to side and softly raise one leg off the floor.
- Side steps: Close your eyes and take 10 steps laterally to one side, then 10 steps to the other.
- Hip kicks: Kick one leg forward, then to the side while maintaining the knee straight. Repeat for the opposite leg.

4. Exercises for Improving Resistance

To enhance muscular strength and endurance, resistance training often consists of lifting weights or pulling against resistance bands. Research discovered that six months of strength training in people with moderate cognitive impairment (MCI) enhanced cognitive ability while also protecting some parts of the brain from further deterioration and atrophy. Notably, the effects were noticeable a year later. Some of these workouts are fairly hard and not recommended for everyone. If your loved one is not physically fit, try altering the exercises to make them less demanding or choosing another activity.

Similarly to balancing exercises, we have written in more depth on how to do these exercises. Several ideas include:

- ☐ Squats Lunges
- ☐ Deadlifts
- ☐ Perform push-ups, chin-ups, planks, and calf raises.

5. Yoga and Tai Chi.

Yoga and Tai-chi provide several advantages for dementia patients, including physical, cognitive, and emotional benefits. Some of them include:

- Increased bone strength, balance, and flexibility.
- Reduced risk of falls
- Improved respiratory, cardiovascular, and circulatory health. Reduced stress.
- Benefits include greater sleep and morning restfulness, reduced risk of sadness and anxiety, and enhanced mood.
- Enhanced cognitive abilities, including memory, attention, awareness, cognition, and language
- Patients new to yoga and tai chi may begin with very basic motions according to their fitness level. YouTube is a great site to get videos of various workouts that are simple to do at home. Some community organizations hold seminars for elderly patients.

6. Seated Exercises.

Seated exercises are a common alternative for people with mobility concerns who may be unable to participate in other types of physical activity.

Patients may safely exercise while sitting in a chair or on the couch.

Ideally, caregivers should participate in the activity, enabling patients to follow along and remain involved. It may also be beneficial to use music to assist you transition from one workout to another.

Some examples of sitting exercises are:

- Holding a ball or a tiny cushion in one hand and spinning at the waist, transferring the ball to the other hand.
- Marching to the beat of the music
- Keep heels on the floor and lean down to tap each pair of toes.
- Lifting arms out in front, then lifting them to the ceiling while wiggling palms and fingers.
- Using the arms of a chair if necessary, attempt to gradually elevate to a standing posture

7. Swimming-pool exercises

Aquatic exercise is an effective kind of physical activity for dementia patients. This is particularly true if individuals have physical injuries, chronic inflammatory disorders like arthritis, or have just had surgery.

Low-impact water workouts are easy on muscles, bones, and joints, allowing patients to increase flexibility and do motions that they would otherwise be unable to accomplish. These activities also boost memory and cognitive function while alleviating depressive symptoms. Participating in an elderly patient program provides an opportunity to mingle and engage with others.

If there are no programs available at a swimming pool near you, patients may participate in water aerobics on their own or with friends and family. Simply notify someone nearby that they are in the pool in case of an emergency.

Some possibilities include:

- Leg swings: While chest deep in water, patients swing one leg at a time, similar to a pendulum. Repeat for both legs.

- ☐ Mini squats: Patients should bend their knees as far as possible, as if sitting in an unseen chair.
- ☐ Marching: Patients may pretend to march on the spot.
- ☐ Arm circles: Patients should be roughly neck deep in the water, making circles with their arms. Begin with tiny circles and progressively expand.

8. Dancing.

Patients may dance anywhere. This practice may be as regimented (by doing certain dance steps) or as unstructured as the patients choose. It's perfect for improving physical, mental, and emotional well-being. Dancing has also been shown in studies to increase strength, muscular function, balance, flexibility, and cardiovascular health.

In addition, dancing to their favorite songs allows them to reflect and recall joyful experiences from previous occasions. Some people may prefer more structured activities, such as dance classes at a local community club.

9. Get Out and About

Patients with dementia might easily get bored at home. Going out for the day may be an excellent opportunity for dementia patients to interact with the world around them and try new activities. It also allows for physical activity, alleviates feelings of despair and anxiety, and reduces disruptive behaviors like hostility and agitation.

Ideas for a day out may include:

- ☐ Go shopping together.
- ☐ Visiting their favorite location in town.
- ☐ Visiting local landmarks or other points of interest
- ☐ Going to the movies or theater.
- ☐ Visit museums or art galleries.
- ☐ Visiting relatives and friends.
- ☐ Caregivers may find it valuable to know ahead of time what services are available. Some venues provide activity days just for dementia patients, such as shortened theater performances or guided tours during quiet hours.

10. Explore nature.

Exploring nature, like going shopping, is an excellent method for dementia people to get out of the home. Your loved one may participate in a wide range of engaging outdoor activities. This is especially beneficial if your loved one liked gardening or had a passion for animals.

Activities to consider are:

- ☐ Gardening (more on this later).
- ☐ Visit a local botanical garden.
- ☐ Going for a stroll or a bike ride in the park
- ☐ Going bird viewing at the nearby nature reserve.
- ☐ Feeding birds or ducks at the pond
- ☐ Simply relax on the lawn and watch the birds.
- ☐ Watching a wildlife documentary (great for rainy days)
- ☐ Nature-based activities are an excellent method for dementia people to be physically active, reduce anxiety, and enjoy themselves. Even a simple stroll in the park may give a variety of sensory stimuli, such as various noises and fragrances, while also improving mood and cognitive performance.

It's critical to ensure that these activities are safe and accessible for dementia patients. Some people may need mobility help or other modifications in order to fully engage in these activities.

11. Help with household chores
Caregivers sometimes struggle to find time to prepare activities for their loved ones. Even just engaging in family activities and assisting with domestic duties may make the patients feel appreciated. The familiar duties might also elicit pleasant memories and spark a discussion. These activities should be customized to the patient's skills so that they feel involved and productive without becoming overwhelmed.

Examples include:

- ☐ Folding clothes, including towels and socks
- ☐ Setting the table.
- ☐ Washing the dishes
- ☐ sweeping the floor.
- ☐ Sorting mail and recycling stuff.

12. Travel and go on vacation
Traveling and going on vacation may be a terrific way to unwind and gain new experiences. It is still absolutely safe for persons with dementia to travel and go on vacation following their diagnosis, although it may need some additional preparation. It may be simpler to go short distances to familiar sites. Long-distance travel may be exhausting and perplexing, particularly for people in the late stages of the condition.

2. Cognitive Activities

Cognitive exercises may preserve (and even increase) cognitive abilities in dementia patients. Any exercise that challenges the brain and helps patients enhance one or more cognitive functions may be classified as cognitive activity. Many studies have shown that individuals with dementia who participate in these activities perform better in all cognitive domains, including memory, thinking, reasoning, attention, problem-solving, and others.

13. Cognitive Games for Therapy

Cognitive stimulation therapy, a key component of dementia treatment at Neural Effects, employs a variety of exercises to assist improve cognitive function and halt the course of symptoms.

Many of these interesting activities do not need any special equipment and are easy adaptable to conduct at home:

- ☐ "Guess the…." game: Variations include guessing the music, flag, state, and more.
- ☐ tale dice: Patients must create a tale based on the images on a die. Patients throw the dice and must come up with an improvised tale.
- ☐ Trivia questions: Patients must answer questions on general knowledge, such as capital cities or notable individuals. This practice enhances cognitive capacities including memory, logic, and problem solving. It also improves communication and social connection.
- ☐ Money: Patients have "money" and need to "buy" various items. This practice helps patients with decision-making when determining what they can afford to buy, as

well as mental math when calculating change after a transaction.

14. Play board or card games.
Board games and card games are excellent ways to spend time together when the weather is bad outdoors or for individuals who have limited mobility. They promote communication and strategic thinking while stimulating memory and cognitive abilities in a pleasant and engaging manner. It is critical to choose a game that the patient can participate in without getting confused or upset.

Examples include:

- ☐ Dominos Bingo
- ☐ UNO, Chute & Ladder, Checkers
- ☐ Solitaire Scrabble Jigsaw puzzles
- ☐ Guess who.
- ☐ Battleship Trivial Pursuit

15. Play Brain Teasers.

Brain teasers, like board games, serve to prevent memory loss and boost cognitive function while also providing chances for social interactions that help patients and caregivers form good emotional connections. For example, research found that completing crossword puzzles on a daily basis prevented cognitive deterioration in dementia patients compared to those who did not participate.

Activities suitable for persons with dementia include:

- ☐ Puzzles include jigsaws and find-a-word challenges.
- ☐ Mazes Brain training apps Sudoku 16. Look at old photos and videos.
- ☐ Looking at old images and videos helps individuals with dementia remember events from the past. These albums include images from their earlier years and might help rekindle treasured memories. It also improves quality of life, cognition, communication skills, and mood, and it's an excellent

opportunity to learn something new about your loved one.

17. Read a book.

Reading, whether fiction or nonfiction, may help people with early dementia improve their communication abilities. This is especially true if your loved one was an ardent reader. Caregivers or other family members may read to people with late-stage dementia who are unable to read for themselves. This is a good activity for youngsters to undertake with their grandparents, for example. If the patient struggles to focus for extended periods of time, try short poetry or picture books that the patient has previously loved. Reading them might evoke memories and spark discussions.

Patients may also listen to their favorite books as audiobooks. This might be a better alternative to television in the evenings or utilized during travel to keep the patient calm.

18. Watch a movie.

Watching movies is another excellent technique to enhance the patient's cognitive abilities and boost emotions of connection with the rest of the family. Each patient has different tastes, although individuals with dementia frequently respond well to films with simple plotlines, such as comedies or musicals.

19. Share jokes and laugh often.
Maintaining a healthy sense of humor may benefit dementia patients. A few years ago, a research titled the SMILE study found that telling patients amusing jokes and making them laugh regularly helped lower levels of anxiety and agitation while also promoting a stronger bond between patient and caregiver. Patients and caregivers may create their own "family" jokes or watch stand-up comedy events, for example.

20. Sort items.
This is an exercise for people with mild to advanced dementia. To improve fine motor skills and cognitive function, patients strive to sort a series of tiny things by color, size, form, and so on. Some

patients may find it amusing to spend some time locating the appropriate things for this game, which may lead to a discussion with the caregiver.

Objects may include:

- ☐ Buttons with colorful beads.
- ☐ Bottle caps
- ☐ Jewelry Cards
- ☐ Rocks
- ☐ Nuts and bolts
- ☐ M&Ms or other colorful candy.

21. Stay in Touch With Friends

Today's technology makes it simple to remain in contact with friends and family, even if they live far apart. This is an excellent chance for dementia patients to contact family members that they may not see as regularly in person. Furthermore, learning to use computers or tablets slows cognitive decline and helps patients stay up with technological advances.

Patients can:

- ☐ Send emails.
- ☐ Use Instant Messages
- ☐ Make video calls (as on Skype and Zoom).
- ☐ Maintain a social media presence (such as Facebook and Instagram).
- ☐ Join online communities.
- ☐ Play online games with others 24. Find Local Support Groups.
- ☐ Joining a local support group is a fantastic opportunity to meet other people with similar diagnoses and participate in a variety of activities. Popular activities include singing, playing musical instruments, acting workshops, arts & crafts, and many more. It's critical to select a group you like. This might include a faith-based group, a reading group, or a creative group, for example. Participating in these organizations may help individuals feel less alone and more like they belong someplace.

3. Sensory Activities

In general, sensory exercises may be quite beneficial in treating cognitive deficits and improving quality of life. These exercises provide patients with various opportunities to engage all five senses, utilizing ordinary things that might elicit happy ideas, memories, or sensations. Sensory exercises are very useful for people who have difficulty connecting with their surroundings.

Sensory activities may involve:

- ☐ Help patients feel protected and calm.
- ☐ Improve the patient's happiness and self-esteem.
- ☐ Improve communication, focus, and other cognitive abilities.
- ☐ Offer chances for sociability.

22. Cooking

For many patients, the kitchen is a familiar space with many pleasant memories. Cooking a dinner for the family might encourage patients to remember and recollect hilarious anecdotes. Cooking is also an excellent sensory exercise, with a variety of aromas, textures, and tastes to enjoy.

Depending on their ability, your loved one may be able to complete a full recipe on their own, or they may need assistance with the more complicated parts. Even if they are in the latter stages of the illness and unable to complete any of the tasks, they gain from watching you cook.

23. Gardening: Many dementia patients valued spending time in their gardens. Gardening, even if it is as simple as caring for little plants inside, is an excellent method to engage the mind and activate all of the senses. Working with plants provides a relaxing impact, elicits memories, and promotes social relationships and wellbeing. It also improves sleep, lowers agitation in dementia patients, and promotes a variety of physical activity, from simple exercise like weeding or raking to more rigorous digging and tree cutting.

From a practical standpoint, if your loved one has difficulty bending, it may be beneficial to invest in elevated beds to make them more accessible from a standing or sitting position.

24. Music

Music is an excellent pastime for persons with dementia. According to studies, music decreases anxiety and sadness while also improving behavior. Music may help even in the late stages of the illness since musical memories are kept after other forms of memory are gone. This is because some of the most important parts of the brain involved in musical memory are often the last to be impacted by the illness.

Music may be utilized in a variety of activities, including:

- ☐ Making playlists for various purposes, such as relaxing before sleep, distracting an agitated patient, or inspiring physical activity.
- ☐ Encourage patients to sing along to music they like. If feasible, patients may desire to dance.
- ☐ Allowing patients to explore with various sounds. Patients may play musical instruments or construct their own using ordinary objects.

25. "Stop and Smell the Roses"
Scents may elicit strong memories since they are
processed in the brain near the memory-controlling
regions. When you go out with your loved one,
encourage them to appreciate familiar aromas, such
as newly cut grass or the perfume of freshly made
bread. It is critical to avoid scents that might evoke
unpleasant memories and induce anxiety.

4. Creative Activities

Patients with dementia gain greatly from creative
activity. Importantly, people in the latter stages of
the illness who may struggle to speak may utilize
creativity to convey their emotions in a nonverbal
fashion. Patients with dementia may sometimes talk
or grin while painting, even if they are unable to do
so regularly.

Furthermore, creative activities provide patients
with a feeling of success and purpose since they
have managed to create something despite the limits
imposed by the sickness. This also reduces stress
and alleviates symptoms of despair and anxiety.

26. Arts & crafts.

Art therapy is one of the most effective therapies for dementia patients. According to studies, it enhances cognitive function, lowers disruptive behavior, and fosters better communication between patients and caregivers. Arts and crafts are also an excellent approach to promote creativity and offer patients a feeling of accomplishment.

Several concepts include:

- ☐ Painting and drawing: Patients do not have to be artists to appreciate using painting and drawing to express themselves artistically. This is their chance to employ big, vibrant colors. Patients in the final stages of the condition sometimes utilize art to communicate nonverbally.
- ☐ Adult coloring books are very beneficial while traveling or while waiting for a doctor's appointment, for example. They're popular for stress alleviation and are widely accessible in craft stores or online.

☐ Crochet and knitting: Even basic projects like a scarf or hat may be quite rewarding to accomplish.

☐ Collages: Patients may make collages by cutting out pictures from magazines or even family photographs. They may choose a topic that reflects their passions, such as cooking, gardening, or vehicles.

☐ Keeping up with seasonal customs, such as constructing Christmas tree decorations, dyeing Easter eggs, or carving a pumpkin for Halloween.

27. Build a Memory Box

Patients with dementia may appreciate putting together a memory box with objects that have particular importance to them. For caregivers, it's an excellent time to interact with the patient and inquire about the products they choose.

The box may include:

☐ Photos of family and dogs
☐ Special souvenirs.

- [ ] Items that remind the patient of their career, such as stationery for someone who used to work in an office or nuts and bolts for a handyman.
- [ ] Items connected to your preferred interests
- [ ] Items relating to your favorite sports team.
- [ ] Items relating to favorite holidays.
- [ ] Items indicating significant events in the patient's life:

28. Create themed boxes.

Patients with dementia, like those who use sensory boxes, may enjoy gathering materials to construct themed boxes. They may return to the box to add more goods or give it as a present to a friend or family.

Some topics to examine include:

- [ ] Garden Box: Patients who were formerly avid gardeners may choose to gather seed packets, little garden tools, stones, or even soil for their gardening bin.

- ☐ dazzling Box: Patients may be looking for dazzling objects around the home, such as jewelry, money, and glitter.
- ☐ Sports lovers may desire to collect caps, keychains, playing cards, and photos of their favorite sports teams.
- ☐ Holiday Box: If patients have just returned from holiday, they may wish to gather souvenirs such as seashells, pebbles, and postcards from their destination.
- ☐ Patients who like painting or sketching may be interested in collecting various craft items such as paint, clay, sponges, and so on.
- ☐ Aromatherapy box: Patients may want to gather various scented oils and lotions to use on different occasions.

Chapter 10

Self-care for Caregivers

When you're giving your all to care for a loved one with dementia, how can you find time and energy to care for yourself?

Even little adjustments may make an impact.

Being a caretaker may be tremendously gratifying, but it can also be stressful. Caring for someone with Alzheimer's or a similar disease requires time and effort. It may be lonely and stressful. You may even feel irritated, which might indicate that you are attempting to take on too much. Making time for self-care is critical. Here are some suggestions that may provide some relief:

- ☐ Request assistance as necessary. This might include requesting family and friends for assistance or contacting local agencies for further care requirements.
- ☐ Eat nutritious meals to stay healthy and active for longer.
- ☐ Join a caregiver support group. Meeting other caregivers allows you to exchange experiences and ideas, which may make you feel less lonely.
- ☐ Take breaks every day. Try brewing a cup of tea or phoning a buddy.
- ☐ Spend time with friends and continue to pursue interests.
- ☐ Exercise as frequently as you can. Try doing yoga or going for a stroll.
- ☐ Try to meditate. According to research, meditation may help with blood pressure, anxiety, despair, and sleeplessness.

☐ Consider obtaining treatment from a mental health expert to deal with stress and worry. Consult your doctor about seeking therapy.

Caregiving may be both physically and emotionally draining. Whether you work in the caregiving industry or care for a loved one, remember to refuel your batteries. Caregivers may also experience financial stress, family strife, and social disengagement. Over time, caregiver stress may cause burnout, which is characterized by irritation, exhaustion, sleep issues, weight gain, feelings of powerlessness or despair, and social isolation.

Caregiver burnout exemplifies how chronic stress may impair both mental and physical health. Chronic stress causes the body to produce stress hormones, which may result in weariness, irritation, a compromised immune system, digestive problems, headaches, pains, and weight gain, particularly around the middle.

Your body has a natural mechanism to battle stress. The parasympathetic nervous system regulates the "relaxation response," which is the counter-stress mechanism. Mind-body therapies such as yoga, tai chi, meditation, and deep relaxation methods may be used to specifically stimulate the relaxation response.

5 Ways to Take Care for oneself as a Caregiver

1. Self-compassion is crucial for self-care.

Being nice to oneself establishes the framework for self-care. Self-compassion is giving yourself credit for the difficult, intricate labor of caring, turning off the self-critical, harsh inner voice, and giving yourself time — even if it's just a few minutes everyday — to look after yourself.

Getting away might be especially difficult when you don't have enough time or energy. What you need to know is that practicing self-care helps the caregiver stay balanced, focused, and productive, which benefits everyone involved.

2. Spend 10 minutes each day practicing basic breath awareness.

One of the most basic deep relaxation methods is breath awareness. Here's something you can try:

- [ ] Assume a comfortable seating posture on a chair or cushion.
- [ ] Shut your eyes and observe your breath.
- [ ] It is normal to have distracting ideas come and go, but just let them pass and gently return your focus to your breath.
- [ ] Inhale gently through your nose for five counts, hold and pause for five counts, then exhale for five counts.
- [ ] Continue for ten minutes. You may replace sentences for the counts, such as:

- [ ] I take in peaceful and calming energies.
- [ ] I stop and let the silent energy settle my body.

3. Engage in a mind-body practice such as yoga, tai chi, meditation, or deep relaxation exercises.

Mind-body activities not only promote physical health, but they also increase awareness and connection between the mind and body. Yoga, deep relaxation methods, and mindfulness meditation may all help to alleviate stress.

4. Prioritize good nutrition and enough sleep.

When attempting to serve others, it is easy to lose sight of your own wants and requirements. Maintaining proper sleep and nourishment is critical to avoiding caregiver burnout. Create a 10-minute evening ritual to get more peaceful sleep. Breathing techniques, meditation, and yoga positions may all be part of your evening regimen. Missing meals may cause anger and exhaustion, so eat regularly planned meals throughout the day.

Nutrition may also help reduce burnout. Chronic stress has been related to increased inflammation in the body, thus it is best to avoid processed meals and foods rich in refined sugars, both of which cause inflammation. Alcohol should be avoided or reduced since it causes inflammation in the body and interferes with sleep quality.

5. Stay socially connected. Find help from local caregiver support organizations.

While keeping social appointments with friends and family might be tough in the midst of medical caregiving, maintaining social relationships is critical for feeling less alienated and preventing burnout.

Realizing that you are not alone and that others are going through similar situations helps you develop self-compassion. Hospitals and community organizations often provide caregiver support groups for families and caregivers.

Conclusion

As we pull the curtains on our investigation of dementia care, we find ourselves on the verge of gaining a better understanding. The chapters that came before this conclusion guided us through the complexities of dementia, a disorder that tries the boundaries of human resilience and compassion. This conclusion is not the end, but rather the beginning—a call to action for caregivers, families, and communities to embrace the path ahead with hope, knowledge, and steadfast support.

Dementia care is an art that combines the scientific and the humanistic. It takes a combination of medical expertise, psychological understanding, and, most importantly, a heart that looks beyond the ailment to the person inside. It is a pledge to respect the individual's history, preferences, and dignity at all stages of their life.

In the face of memory loss and cognitive decline, the value of human interaction becomes even more apparent. The delicate touch gives comfort, careful listening provides peace, and shared laughter creates delight. These ties are lifelines for both the person with dementia and their caretakers.

Dementia care goes beyond the house; it is a communal concern. Societies must respond to the problem by providing inclusive settings that help people with dementia and their families. From dementia-friendly companies to governmental policies that emphasize care, the community plays a critical role in establishing a society that values and cares for its older population.

Caregivers are the hidden heroes of dementia care, often prioritizing the needs of their loved ones before their own. This book acknowledges the physical, mental, and spiritual toll that caring may have. It serves as a reminder that caregivers, like patients, need care, support, and time to recover. They must be seen, recognized, and respected for the significant job they do.

While there is presently no cure for dementia, the promise of science and innovation serves as a light of hope. Scientists across the globe are working feverishly to unlock the secrets of the brain, hoping for discoveries that may one day change the landscape of dementia care. This book supports their quest, praising every step gained in knowledge and therapy.

Looking forward, we envisage a world where dementia care is characterized by compassion, creativity, and diversity. A future in which caregivers are supported, dementia patients are treated with dignity, and communities are prepared to offer the necessary resources and support.

Allow us to keep the lessons acquired from these pages with us as we go on our next trip. Let us remember that at the center of dementia care is the chance to demonstrate the finest of what it is to be human—to care, love, and connect on the most profound levels. Let us go ahead determined to make a difference, to enhance the lives of individuals suffering from dementia, and to leave a legacy of care for future generations.